If You Find a Lump in Your Breast...

MARTHA McLEAN

with the assistance of
JACQUELINE J. STRUTHERS, M.D.
General and Thoracic Surgeon

BULL PUBLISHING COMPANY, *Palo Alto*

Bull Publishing Company
P.O. Box 208
Palo Alto, California 94302

ISBN 0-915950-47-2
Library of Congress Catalogue Number 80-69209

IF YOU FIND A LUMP IN YOUR BREAST..

Contents

Why This Booklet

My mastectomy was in January 1976. A small "shadow" appeared on a mammogram, and all of a sudden I found myself in a strange world—with new language, unknown threats, and seemingly urgent deadlines.

I was lucky.

There was a careful and unhurried explanation by a stranger—"my surgeon." I heard some of it. But much, I now realize, was blocked out by my emotions and by questions of my own that kept welling up in my mind as I tried to listen.

These are some of those questions, answered by that surgeon. I think they may be some of the same questions you have. *They are not intended to take the place of your own questions to your own doctor; they are the things I wish I'd understood better before my surgery.*

I have learned that the answers aren't all in yet on treating cancer of the breast—therefore, there are controversies. Within the medical profession, there are differences of opinion. We are left with many questions which do not yet have a "right" answer.

But the answers are coming in. New studies are changing modes of treatment. What I write today may be changed, almost by tomorrow. This is good; progress is being made.

REMEMBER: This is a field undergoing constant change, with new developments which may supersede present forms of diagnosis and treatment.

There is a role for some of you, as patients, to participate in helping to find the answers to questions so important to us and our daughters. You may have the opportunity—as I did—to take part in the nationwide studies funded by the National Cancer Institute to compare different forms of breast cancer treatment.

Dr. Bernard Fisher, chairman of the test program, emphasizes that these "clinical trials" comparing different combinations of surgery, radiation and drugs, are an "ethical facet of medicine and do not represent experimenting in any derogatory sense."

Breast cancer is a scientific problem, a biological problem. If we are to obtain the badly-needed answers to these remaining problems, participation in these carefully monitored studies is necessary to prove the ultimate worth of different forms of treatment.

If you are interested in taking part in current treatment trials, you can phone the National Cancer Institute, toll-free, at (800) 638-6694. Travel and treatment, including reconstruction, may be without charge for some trials. Be sure you understand the commitment involved and your rights. Or you may phone Dr. Fisher at (412) 624-2672.

We shouldn't look for miraculous or sudden breakthroughs, but we can expect progress toward more and more effective treatment.

I have found a new appreciation of how different we all are, as women, as patients. I personally believe that we have a right·to full information. There *are* choices, and many of us feel a need to participate in making those choices.

"Patient participation" is a new and difficult role for us all—patients and physicians. I also recognize that some women would rather not share in this responsibility, and that should be their privilege.

In recent years mastectomy has been brought out into the open, and many old fears have been dispelled. As an informed patient, you can help do the same for your friends and family.

After mastectomy, you can and should expect to be basically the same woman you always have been. You should be able to do the same things—wear the same clothes—enjoy the same activities as before.

Dr. Struthers told me: "Don't let cancer change your life...except perhaps to find a deeper appreciation of those around you and the beauty of the world we live in."

Martha McLean
1980

Diagnosis

What are the chances that a lump is cancer?

Most breast lumps are not malignant.

On an overall basis, 75 to 80 percent—or more—are benign; but only a physician can make the diagnosis.

On an individual basis, the possibility of cancer varies with each woman, depending on several factors: your age and family history, your menstrual status, what the physician's examination of your breast indicates, and what breast X-ray (mammogram or xerogram) shows.

Your risk increases somewhat if there is breast cancer in your family, especially if your mother or sister had it, and perhaps if breast cancer is present in your father's family.

You also join a higher risk group if you are over the age of 40, or have had no children, or had your children after the age of about 30, or started to menstruate before the age of 12. If you have had radiation treatment for mastitis (inflammation of the breast) in the past, an annual, careful check-up by your doctor is wise.

A lump is the most common sign of possible cancer of the breast. Other changes that should alert you to see a doctor are discharge from one nipple, a dimpling of the flesh, an eczema-like irritation or a change of color of the skin—in short, any change from the usual appearance or feel of your breasts. In examining your breasts, you and the physician should also check for lumps in the underarm area.

How can the doctor tell if a lump is benign or malignant?

There are a number of ways a physician makes a diagnosis; usually a combination of methods is used.

In many cases, the physician is able to tell with considerable accuracy whether a lump is benign or malignant by *palpation*—that is, examining with his fingers. But some lumps cannot be precisely identified in this way. Sometimes a physician will use *transillumination* (showing a bright light through the affected area of the breast) to find out whether the lump is solid or filled with fluid. If fluid can be withdrawn through a needle ("aspiration" or "fine needle biopsy"), the lump is a cyst and usually benign. However, as a wise precaution, it is sent to a laboratory to check for cancer cells.

Thermography measures the extra heat given off by diseased cells; it is now little used because it is not accurate enough to be really helpful.

Meanwhile, the search continues for a method of diagnosis which does not involve X-ray or surgery. So far X-ray is still the most reliable method we have, aside from biopsy.

Breast X-ray is a valuable, though not infallible, guide. Either *mammography* or *xeromammography* is considered to be 60-85 percent accurate, depending on the experience of the technician, the radiologist who reads the X-ray, and the quality of the "picture."

Though correct in most cases, occasionally a breast X-ray can be either false-positive (X-ray indicates cancer, though lump proves later to be benign) or false-negative (X-ray suggests that the lump is benign, but it later turns out to be malignant).

Mammography sometimes shows calcifications, which the doctor cannot see or feel. Many of these prove to be harmless, but approximately one-third are associated with cancer.

Even when the X-ray shows probable malignancy, a biopsy is the most accurate means of arriving at a final diagnosis.

In deciding whether a patient should or should not have surgery for a breast lump, the physician's initial judgment is based on information from personal history, clinical examination, and tests such as mammography. But for a definitive diagnosis, a biopsy is required. By removing all or a portion of the lump surgically and examining it under a microscope, it is possible to determine whether cancer cells are present. More about this later.

How much risk is there in having a mammogram or xerogram?

Both of these are X-rays of the breast, using a special technique to bring out certain signs of cancer in the lump. Both are painless and take less than an hour.

A mammogram is the usual X-ray type film; a xerogram uses a special Xerox technique (xeroradiography) which produces a picture with blue lines on a white background or white lines on a blue background.

The results from both can be available immediately, so any delay in learning the results depends on the time it takes for a radiologist to read them and report to your physician. Some radiologists prefer the film-type mammogram; others, the xerogram. There is considered to be little or no difference in accuracy.

The risk of radiation from these exams has been a frequent topic in the press. The physician must weigh the risks of such radiation against the risk of not having the information such X-rays can give. Age and family history are taken into consideration in deciding who needs breast X-ray.

Dr. Philip Strax, well-known breast cancer specialist who is medical director of the Guttman Breast Diagnostic Institute in New York, states: "With modern techniques, the X-ray dose can be and has been cut so low that risk is negligible even on a periodic basis compared to the potential benefit."

Dr. Strax' guidelines, which agree with guidelines revised in 1977 by a study committee of the National Cancer Institute and the American Cancer Society,* are as follows:

Under age 35, women should not have mammograms routinely unless there are good reasons for this exam as determined by the physician, such as abnormal symptoms or signs. Between 35 and 49, women without symptoms should not have routine mammographic examination unless they have a personal history of breast cancer or breast cancer in the immediate family (mother or sister). Over the age of 50, there is a definite benefit from annual mammography, whether there are symptoms or not.

---

*The American Cancer Society guidelines are reprinted at p. 78.

ACS-NCI standards specify one rad or less per exam: you should ask about the machine, and when it was last checked, *before* making an appointment for an exam. The risk is not in a single exposure, but the possible cumulative effect of repeated exams has been the focus of concern. Some authorities feel that there is no minimum safe level of irradiation, but the risk does get smaller as the dose gets smaller.

It should be stressed that the mammography controversy concerns only *routine or screening* use of mammography for women with no symptoms. For women of any age in which there is a suspected breast cancer, mammography is an acceptable and valuable part of a complete diagnostic work-up.

How is a biopsy performed and what does it show?

A biopsy is the surgical removal of a piece of tissue for examination. This may sound much more ominous than it is. It is a simple procedure that can be performed under either local or general anesthesia and *usually is not painful.* Biopsies can be done as a hospital "in-patient," as an "out-patient," or in a doctor's office.

The incision is usually made right over the lump or around the nipple. The lump is totally removed in most cases (excisional biopsy); but if it is too large, only a portion may be removed (incisional biopsy).

The purpose of the biopsy is to obtain tissue to put under the microscope in order to make a definite diagnosis. But this is also an important decision point.

Before a biopsy is done, the decision must be made between immediate or delayed treatment, in case the biopsy shows cancer. If you and your physician decide on immediate treatment—the one-step procedure—surgery is performed directly following the biopsy while you are still under anesthesia. If delayed treatment is chosen—the two-step procedure—just the biopsy is performed and you wait to make the decision on treatment. Based on information from the biopsy and further tests, the decision is then made on whether mastectomy or another form of treatment is best suited to your individual case.

Which approach is best for you should be thoroughly discussed at this time, if possible with a "team" of doctors—your own physician and cancer specialists (e.g., a surgical oncologist and a radiation oncologist). (See page 16 for more information on the one-step and two-step procedures.)

When making arrangements for a surgical biopsy, you should ask to have an ER assay performed. (See page 29)

Another form of biopsy is wide-needle biopsy, in which tissue is withdrawn through a hollow needle inserted into the lump. It can be performed in the physician's office; for small lumps, however, its usefulness is limited because of the risk that the needle can miss its mark. Negative needle biopsies have no significance, because an adequate sample may not have been obtained. However, a positive needle biopsy is as useful diagnostically as one in which all or part of the cancer is surgically removed.

For some lumps, the physician is able to aspirate the lump, that is, withdraw fluid through a needle. Such lumps are usually benign, but should be carefully watched and checked.

What are the main kinds of breast cancer?

There are many kinds of breast cancer, the number depending on how you classify them. A majority occur in the ducts—the tubes which carry the milk. A list of the principal types of breast cancer is included in the section, "Understanding the Language" under *Breast Cancer*, page 62. There are many sub-groups within these categories, some with almost untranslatable names. All, except sarcoma, come under the umbrella of "mammary carcinoma."

Do men get breast cancer?

Men do get breast cancer, mostly older men, but it is very rare. There will be 100 breast cancers in women for each breast cancer in men.

Where can I get medical help?

For some women even deciding where to start is a problem. If you find a lump in your breast, please don't wait and wonder and worry about it. Since a lump is more likely to be benign than malignant, you owe it to yourself and your family to find out the cause rather than to worry—probably needlessly.

Most women go first to their own family physician or gynecologist. If your doctor feels a biopsy is needed, he usually will recommend a surgeon. For your own peace of mind, this should be a person with whom you feel at ease to ask questions and receive satisfying answers. If you have doubts, you should ask for a second medical opinion.

If you do not have a personal physician, you can phone your county medical society for physician referral. Also a phone call to your local American Cancer Society (ACS) office should reach someone who knows the various facilities in your community or nearby, such as community hospitals that have "Approved Cancer Programs." These hospitals meet criteria established by the American College of Surgeons and can provide you with the names of qualifed physicians on their staffs. If finances are a problem, people at ACS also can advise you about possibilities for assistance.

Cancer Facts and Figures, published by the American Cancer Society, has a list of the comprehensive cancer centers funded by the National Cancer Institute. Jane Brody's book, *You Can Fight Cancer and Win* (see page 56), contains a section on cancer services, which includes a list of hospitals with approved cancer programs as well as the comprehensive cancer centers. Some of the centers have toll-free information services. Even if your community does not have cancer specialists (oncologists), a communications network with cancer centers across the nation makes consultation with such specialists available to all doctors.

Many hospitals have social workers who are trained to help with emotional stress, family concerns, financial and other problems. Some nurses also have received special training for cancer care and can be of real help to you in finding answers to concerns you may have. In some areas the American Cancer Society has volunteers who have had a mastectomy, or breast reconstruction, who will visit with you before surgery, with the permission of your physician.

As important as "where do I start?" is "when?" The answer is: Don't panic, but get professional help as soon as you suspect a lump.

There is no need for frantic action. But much of the responsibility is on your own shoulders—about 95 percent of the time a lump is found by the woman herself. If all women would get early treatment, chances of cure would improve greatly.

Also, always remember that early detection is your best protection against cancer of the breast. So acting as soon as you find any suspicious symptoms is definitely to your advantage.

Treatment

How is cancer of the breast treated?

The major forms of cancer treatment are surgery, radiation and chemotherapy; immunotherapy is a separate experimental type of therapy, which utilizes a vaccine to mobilize the body's natural immune system. In breast cancer, as in other forms of cancer, combined therapies are often used. Presently much study is going on to determine which treatment combination will produce the best results with least damage.

For many years surgery has been the primary treatment for breast cancer. Biopsy is a form of surgery, and in that sense treatment almost always begins with this essentially diagnostic form of surgery, to remove the lump (or, if very large, a portion of it) to find out whether cancer is present. The various forms of breast surgery will be discussed later.

Radiation destroys cancer cells locally by means of high energy rays, such as X-ray. Chemotherapy is treatment with drugs which kill cancer cells throughout the body.

More and more, cancer of the breast is considered a "multidisciplinary" disease, with each form of treatment—surgery, radiation, and chemotherapy—having a role. In large medical centers it may be treated by a team of physicians rather than the surgeon alone. Your case may be discussed by several specialists at "tumo. boards," available at more than 1,000 hospitals in the United States.

What is meant by one-step and two-step procedures?

In a one-step procedure, a biopsy is done under general anesthesia in the hospital. The surgeon removes the lump, closes the wound, sends the tissue to the pathologist for immediate examination of the "frozen section," and waits in the operating room for the report. (See pages 62 and 66 for definitions of biopsy and frozen section.) Under the pathologist's microscope the frozen section can show one of three things:

1) That the lump is definitely benign.

2) That the pathologist is not sure whether it is cancer and recommends waiting for the "permanent section"—this procedure and its report take from 24 hours to several days.

3) That the lump is definitely cancer of the breast. In this case, the surgeon proceeds immediately with the previously agreed upon form of surgery.

In a two-step procedure, treatment is delayed. After the biopsy, the woman is informed she has cancer, treatment methods are discussed with her, and a plan is developed.

Some surgeons believe that a biopsy can be done on an out-patient basis under local anesthesia, without undue risk of the cancer spreading or danger from the delay between the biopsy and further treatment. A National Cancer Institute panel of specialists agreed in June 1979 that a two-step procedure should be used in most cases.

What are the advantages and disadvantages of the one-step and two-step procedures?

ADVANTAGES OF A ONE-STEP PROCEDURE:

The need for two separate operations—and possibly two general anesthesias—is eliminated. For many, there is the psychological advantage of having the tumor already out by the time you find out if it's cancer.

With an adequate doctor-patient relationship, the options are clearly explained, and you can take part in an informed decision on the appropriate surgery before the biopsy.

Other possible advantages are that your chance of wound infection may be less with the one-step procedure, and some (though probably few) surgeons feel that the possibility of spread of cancer cells is greater with the two-step procedure.

The one-step procedure is generally indicated in cases where the surgeon is almost certain that the tumor is malignant.

DISADVANTAGES OF A ONE-STEP PROCEDURE:

The doctor must go into the full details of a mastectomy before the biopsy: the incision, the various kinds of surgery, the possible risks, and how you will look post-op. This is not only time-consuming for both the doctor and the patient, but may be an unnecessarily frightening experience to go through since you may be one of the 75–80 percent who end up having just a biopsy.

Also, because "staging" to determine the extent of the cancer is seldom done before surgery in the one-step procedure, surgery may not be as limited as it could be. Some medical experts believe that lesser surgery is called for if tests such as liver and bone scans show that cancer has spread to other parts of the body.

ADVANTAGES OF A TWO-STEP PROCEDURE:

Some women can accept the idea of having just the biopsy with less apprehension. When done under local anesthesia, the procedure is considered minor surgery, taking less than an hour and not necessitating an overnight hospital stay.

After the biopsy, with the knowledge that she does have cancer, the patient can take part more objectively in selecting the treatment best suited to her needs. On the basis of the permanent section (see page 70), she and the physician know a great deal more about the kind of breast cancer she has and can decide on the treatment or combination of treatments required. In most cases the biopsy has removed the entire lump, so she has the reassurance that the bulk of the cancer is gone.

For some women the interval between biopsy and surgery provides needed time for thinking, planning, psychological preparation for herself and her family, getting home and job organized, etc.

After the biopsy, further tests or "staging" can be done to determine whether the cancer has spread to other parts of the body. If the cancer has spread, some surgeons now feel that a lesser surgical procedure is needed, with chemotherapy or radiotherapy started early to treat cancer cells which have spread to other organs.

Biopsy as an out-patient is also less expensive than the hospital stay required for the one-step procedure.

DISADVANTAGES OF A TWO-STEP PROCEDURE:

The psychological aspects of having to wait, several days to possibly a week, between biopsy and definitive treatment for breast cancer could be a real problem for some women.

The possibility of spread of the tumor during this interval should not have much bearing on whether you choose the one or two-step procedure. Studies have shown that survival is not affected by waiting up to six weeks following biopsy.

The two anesthesias needed for the two-step procedure are considered to be a problem in some cases. Unless the lump is large, some surgeons prefer to do a biopsy under general anesthesia because of the possibility of not being able to feel or identify a small lump after a local anesthesia is injected. In these cases, the disadvantages of the two general anesthesias must be weighed against the advantages of the preoperative "work-up" or "staging" between biopsy and surgery to determine the extent of the cancer. Also, in a large breast, some tumors may be too deeply located to remove under local anesthesia.

What are the various kinds of breast surgery and how do the scars look?

Remember that no surgical site is pleasant to look at right after the operation. However, with healing, there will be a great improvement in appearance, and most scars become a lot less obvious as time passes. For an indication of the different types of incisions, see page 22.

The object of surgery is to remove malignant tissue from its original site and adjacent areas into which it may have spread. The extent of the surgery is another subject of controversy in breast cancer treatment. The National Cancer Institute is in the process of conducting studies (clinical trials called "protocols") to compare the effectiveness of different surgical procedures, both alone and in combination with other forms of treatment (radiation and chemotherapy), but it will take many years to get valid answers.

The principal kinds of surgery performed for breast cancer are described below, but you should be aware that the procedures vary somewhat from surgeon to surgeon. You may wish to discuss with your surgeon what he specifically plans to do and how the incision can least affect your personal preferences in such matters as swimming and clothing choices.

RADICAL MASTECTOMY
(Also Called Classical or Halsted Mastectomy)

Through a vertical or horizontal incision, the entire breast including the nipple is removed, along with the underlying major and minor pectoral muscles and the lymph nodes in the armpits and outer chest wall. Skin grafting may be necessary, and a hollow area is left near the armpit under the collarbone, where the muscles are removed. This is the operation surgeons preferred until several years ago, but many have now changed to the *modified radical* because studies have shown that cure rates are about the same as for the classical radical. However, some tumors close to or invading the chest muscles are not suited for a modified radical.

EXTENDED RADICAL MASTECTOMY

This is a radical mastectomy combined with removal of the internal mammary nodes under the breastbone. This procedure is not generally done, but may be indicated in a younger woman whose cancer is in the inner quadrants of the breast (toward the center of the body).

MODIFIED RADICAL MASTECTOMY
(Total mastectomy with axillary dissection)

Through a vertical or horizontal incision, the entire breast, including the nipple and the axillary lymph nodes, are removed. This is essentially the Halsted radical mastectomy, with the important difference that the *pectoral muscles (one or both)* are saved. With the muscles left in place, use of the arm is usually regained more readily, and swelling of the arm after surgery (lymphedema) is less common.

In addition, the removal of nodes may be less extensive than with the Halsted radical, as it can be more difficult to remove them when the pectoral muscles are left intact. Techniques vary with the modified radical; the upper third of the axillary (armpit) nodes may remain, but many surgeons remove nodes to the top of the armpit.

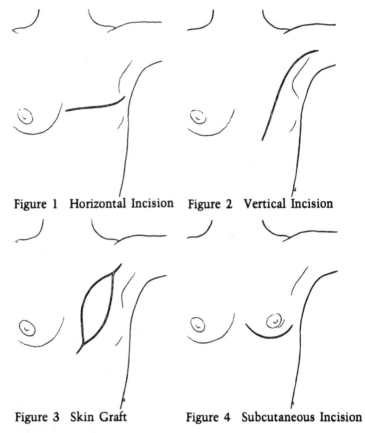

Figure 1   Horizontal Incision   Figure 2   Vertical Incision

Figure 3   Skin Graft   Figure 4   Subcutaneous Incision

TYPES OF INCISIONS

These sketches will give you a general idea of the location of incisions used in breast surgery. Some may be longer or shorter, higher or lower, depending on individual differences among patients and the surgeon's technique. Horizontal or vertical incisions (Figures 1 and 2) are generally used for radical, modified radical, and simple mastectomy. The skin graft (Figure 3) is used in some cases of radical surgery, but is not needed for all. In a subcutaneous mastectomy, the incision is usually under the breast (Figure 4) and the nipple remains. See pages 20-25 for explanations of different forms of surgery.

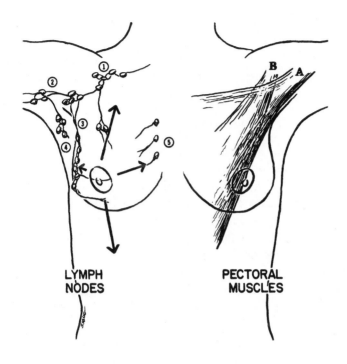

THE LYMPH SYSTEM AND
MAJOR CHEST MUSCLES

Arrows on the left side of the sketch show routes of possible spread of cancer cells in the breast to the lymph nodes. The nodes are part of the lymph system which carries waste from all body tissues and also carries the fluid of the immune system. The nodes can destroy many of the cancer cells which reach them, but sometimes are not able to trap all of them, and cancer cells can then be carried to other parts of the body. The lymph nodes of the breast area are 1) clavicular nodes, 2) upper axillary nodes, 3) middle axillary nodes, 4) lower axillary nodes, and 5) internal mammary nodes. The muscles on the right side of the sketch are the pectoral muscles—pectoralis major (A) and pectoralis minor (B), which are removed in radical surgery.

For early breast cancer, a panel of experts convened by the National Cancer Institute in June 1979 agreed that this procedure (referred to as total mastectomy combined with axillary dissection) is now accepted "standard procedure."

TOTAL OR SIMPLE MASTECTOMY

Through a vertical or horizontal incision, all breast tissue, including the nipple, is removed. This is the same as a modified radical mastectomy, except the axillary nodes are *not* removed. Although in the past most surgeons inspected the axilla for enlarged or hard nodes, microscopic examination of the nodes was usually not performed; thus, the physician did not know whether the cancer had spread to the nodes (an indication that further treatment might be needed).

However, in many cases planned for simple or partial mastectomy, surgeons now "sample" some lymph nodes before surgery to check for malignancy, and if cancer has spread to the nodes, radiation or a modified radical mastectomy is substituted.

SUBCUTANEOUS MASTECTOMY

Through an incision beneath the breast, most breast tissue, including the axillary tail up to the armpit, is removed. Most breast skin, including the nipple and areola, and a small button of breast tissue under the nipple remains. (Figure 4, page 22)

Subcutaneous mastectomy is usually performed as a *preventive* measure for women who have a strong history of breast cancer in the family, or benign breast disease. A plastic implant may be inserted at the time of surgery or later. Some surgeons have serious doubts about this operation in the treatment of cancer, based on problems of possible recurrence on the chest wall and the fact that too few cases have been treated by this method with a sufficient follow-up interval to be evaluated.

LIMITED PROCEDURES

For a *partial mastectomy*, the tumor and a wide segment of surrounding breast tissue are removed. For *lesser surgeries*, such as lumpectomy, tylectomy and segmentectomy, the tumor and a small amount of the surrounding tissue are removed, retaining other breast tissue and skin. (You may hear a number of other terms for these lesser procedures, such as "segmental resection," "local excision" and "wide excision.") The position of the incision in these procedures depends upon the location of the tumor. While the incision could be around the nipple, it is more likely to be elsewhere, over the tumor.

If the cancer is small, with well-defined edges, removing the lump followed by careful and consistent watching, can be an option. However, this is a calculated risk because there is no way to know definitely whether the cancer has spread to the nodes unless the axillary nodes are biopsied or removed. Some very small cancers have been found to have spread to the nodes.

Also, as almost one-third of breast cancers are multicentric (microscopic cancer cells may exist undetected in other portions of the breast), radiation or chemotherapy or both are often recommended in combination with lesser surgery.

When is radiation therapy used?

Distinctions between the different uses of radiation must be understood to help clear the confusion about its use in relation to breast cancer. First, low-energy X-ray is used as a diagnostic tool for screening. Second, high energy X-rays, including gamma rays, are used for treatment. Treatment by radiation takes several forms: primary, as the principal therapy; preventive or prophylactic to destroy possible cells at the surgery site (this is generally referred to as "adjuvant therapy"—see page 28), and as palliative treatment to reduce pain of advanced disease.

Radiation as primary treatment for breast cancer is applied externally by cobalt or linear accelerator machines to a carefully marked area on the chest. The remainder of the body is shielded for protection. Sometimes, in addition to external treatment, radiation is used internally by placing radioactive implants in the breast, usually under general anesthesia. These implants, called "interstitial," are in thin rods and provide an additional local radiation boost while the patient stays in the hospital two or three days. They are removed before the patient is discharged. The effect on the texture of the breast varies from very little to considerable.

Lumpectomy with radiation therapy has been used for some 30 years, but it has not yet been commonly employed as primary treatment. In the past decade, considerable experience has been gained with this form of treatment by physicians and faculty at such institutions as the University of Southern California and Harvard and their affiliated hospitals. However, these

procedures require sophisticated equipment and special-
ized medical staff which may not be available in all
areas of the country. Many factors enter into selecting
this treatment option, such as the type and size of the
lump, age and general health.

The National Cancer Institute started clinical trials
several years ago, comparing modified radical surgery
with lumpectomy plus radiation to the breast and
nodes. While preliminary results are encouraging, many
physicians feel that more time must pass before we can
know for sure whether survival rates are as good with
this treatment as with more traditional surgery.

The long-term effects of radiation are not clearly
known, and some women experience side-effects such
as nausea and weakness, although better machines and
techniques now eliminate or minimize side-effects.
However, this form of treatment can offer a real psychological plus—the breast is almost always preserved in
cancers up to the size of a walnut. It offers an alternative
for women who refuse to have a mastectomy, especially
in early cases. The hope is that more women will be
willing to seek treatment earlier if they can avoid a
mastectomy without undue risk.

What is adjuvant therapy?

Adjuvant therapy for breast cancer is secondary or
additional treatment given to assist or increase the
effectiveness of the primary treatment—most commonly surgery. This is usually applied before there is
evidence of recurrence of tumor, to increase chances of
cure.

Most doctors feel that by the time some breast cancers are detected, they *may* have already spread beyond the area that can be removed surgically and may not be found by physical examination, X-ray or scan. Such spread occurs via the lymphatic and blood systems to such organs as the bones, lung, liver and brain. In addition, even the best of surgeons could leave microscopic cancer cells behind on the chest wall. These residual cells can give rise to a 5 to 20 percent incidence of chest wall recurrences, depending on the size and extent of the breast cancer.

There are three types of adjuvant therapy for breast cancer: radiation therapy, chemotherapy (which includes hormonal therapy), and immunotherapy. Surgery and radiation are localized treatments. Chemotherapy and immunotherapy are systemic treatments; that is, they go throughout the body. Radiation therapy and chemotherapy can produce partial or complete regressions of advanced tumors. However, their effectiveness when used as adjuvant therapy remains to be proven.

ADJUVANT RADIATION THERAPY

Radiation therapy as adjuvant therapy was, until recent years, the standard form of therapy for most patients with positive axillary nodes (nodes with demonstrated cancer cells) and is considered a proven type of treatment by many physicians. Many doctors believe there is still a place for post-operative radio-therapy if the lump is in the inside quadrants of the breast, or if many axillary lymph nodes are involved with tumor.

Others believe that post-operative radiation does not improve survival rates; they feel that radiation decreases a patient's tolerance of chemotherapy and point to studies indicating that the survival rate is not improved by radiation. Radiation does, however, reduce the risk of a local recurrence of cancer on the chest wall or in the axilla and probably will continue to be used in special cases as a type of adjuvant therapy.

ADJUVANT CHEMOTHERAPY

Adjuvant chemotherapy using one or a combination of drugs is presently under extensive study. Preliminary reports are encouraging, and for patients with positive nodes, surgery is often followed by chemotherapy. Thus far, impressive protection has been shown for pre-menopausal women, and studies are still in progress to determine the role of adjuvant therapy for post-meno-pausal women.

The possible side effects of chemotherapy, such as nausea and temporary loss of hair, vary according to the drugs used and each individual's tolerance. Treatment is tailored to each case—we now know much more about the drugs and dosage, and also have newer drugs—and most people can continue to go about their daily tasks while undergoing chemotherapy.

Many questions remain to be answered, and more years must pass before we know the long-term effects of chemotherapy—how useful it will prove or what its possible side-effects may be.

It is now recommended that before a biopsy, arrangements should be made for an estrogen receptor test *(ER assay)*. This test can be done only on tissue taken at the time of biopsy or surgery and can indicate whether *hormone (endocrine) therapy,* a form of chemotherapy, might be helpful immediately as adjunctive therapy, or later if cancer reappears.

The basis of this test is that some breast cancers are

dependent on estrogen for their growth. They are ER positive. Eliminating estrogen does not help in cases of cancers without estrogen receptors (which are ER negative), but about two thirds of patients with positive ER assays are helped by hormone therapy. Thus the results of the ER assay can provide valuable information for decision on future treatment, and you should request this test before a biopsy.

In hormone therapy, the level of estrogen in the body is changed. This is done either by surgically removing estrogen-producing organs such as the ovaries under general anesthetic, or by administering large doses of hormones or anti-estrogen drugs, such as tamoxifen, which has few or mild side-effects.

IMMUNOTHERAPY

Immunotherapy is experimental, and used only by certain medical centers which are conducting "trials" to determine whether it is effective. The purpose of immunotherapy is to stimulate the immune system to combat cancer cells. (See *Immunotherapy*, page 67)

New information keeps coming in concerning both radiation and chemotherapy. Therefore, you may wish to seek advice from medical oncologists or radiation oncologists, who keep up-to-date in this field.

In the long term, as we learn more about the behavior of breast cancer, lesser surgery combined with radiation or chemotherapy may turn out to be an alternative for larger numbers of women.

At present, however, we have no way of knowing which women will have recurrence of breast cancer and are in need of adjuvant treatment. Those whose cancer has spread to axillary nodes or with large, ulcerated

tumors are at higher risk of recurrent disease and probably should have adjuvant treatment.

Helene Brown, past president of the California Division of the American Cancer Society, summed it up:
"Breast cancer is a contradictory, complex disease that
cannot be fit into tables and slots. You should choose
your physician well, one that you can talk with, and
take your chance on 'educated opinion.'"

What is prophylactic mastectomy?

Prophylactic or preventive mastectomy is a mastectomy done when no evidence of malignancy is present
in the breast operated on. Some physicians now recommend preventive mastectomy when it is thought there
is a higher-than-average risk that a malignancy will
develop—such as women with a strong family history
of breast cancer or troublesome cystic disease.

Prophylactic mastectomy may be considered for a
woman who has had surgery on one breast for cancer,
and later the other breast is removed as a preventive
measure because of higher risk factors, such as family
history, benign cystic disease, and the tendency of some
breast cancer to develop in both breasts. Or in some
cases both breasts may be removed at the same time, if
risk factors are high, and especially if a woman is
emotionally upset by the idea of possible cancer.

The loss of both breasts is more easily handled by
some women than the continuing threat of cancer, and
rather than undergo the strain of repeated biopsies, they
prefer bilateral mastectomy. There still seems to be
some disagreement about whether the risk of breast

cancer is greater among women with benign breast disease, so other factors such as family history and emotional well-being should also figure into a decision about preventive mastectomy.

A prophylactic mastectomy may be performed as either a subcutaneous or simple (see page 24) procedure, most commonly the former. Reconstruction can be done at the same time or at a later time.

Cancer management today is becoming increasingly individualized with respect to both diagnostic procedures and treatment. Early detection is followed by precise staging of the disease and the use of more than one kind of therapy, often in combination.

The American Cancer Society
"Cancer Facts & Figures, 1982"

Personal Concerns

What is "informed consent"?

The law requires that doctors inform their patients of any procedure, either diagnostic or treatment, that might be necessary.

The information necessary for such consent includes an explanation of the proposed procedure and any portions that may be experimental, potential hazards and complications, a description of discomfort and risk, a description of benefits, *possible alternative procedures*, an offer to answer any questions, and an explanation that the person is free to withdraw consent and discontinue the recommended care at any time.

You should sign a consent form only after you are satisfied on the above points, and only when the exact procedure you and the surgeon have agreed upon is specified on the form.

How soon should I make a decision?

That is a difficult question to answer. Once a breast tumor can be felt, it has probably been growing for a long time, perhaps many years. So taking a few weeks to make a decision shouldn't present a serious risk. This is a time when careful evaluation and investigation, leading to careful decision-making, are wise.

However, some doctors prefer that, once discovered, a lump be removed as soon as this can be conveniently arranged. Timing can depend, too, on the findings of the clinical exam, mammogram or xerogram, and in the case of the two-step procedure, what the biopsy shows. Some patients wish to have the surgery as soon as possible; others need time to adjust and digest the information they have received. These patients should be carefully counseled by their doctor that unless the cancer is an aggressive type, waiting a reasonable time—four to six weeks—can be helpful and not harmful.

Can I change my mind?

Some patients feel "locked in" once they reach a decision. As stated above, you can change your mind at any time—even after you have signed the consent form—but you should understand the possible consequences of doing so. The important thing to remember is that before medication or surgery—preferably sooner, of course—you should discuss all the alternatives with your physician and should understand the possible courses of action.

How much will surgery hurt? Will chemotherapy or radiation make me feel sick? How long will I live?

These are questions all of us ask, perhaps aloud, perhaps only in our own minds. But there is no single answer that fits all of us. We are all individuals, and each reacts in her own way.

General health, age, psychological make-up—all have a bearing on these questions. It is important also to understand that cancers are different; they are found at different stages and behave unpredictably. Treatment depends on all these variables and must be tailored to each individual person.

If you have not been in a hospital for some years, you will be pleased to find that new techniques, better anesthesias, antibiotics and other improvements reduce pain and help speed recovery. You may find yourself up and walking sooner than you thought possible.

As for the effects of chemotherapy and radiation, these vary according to the drugs and dosage, which, again, are tailored to your individual needs and tolerance. Hospitalization is not usually required for either, and most women are able to continue their usual daily work while under treatment.

And finally, always remember: No one—including doctors—can or should say how long anyone will live. Our best kind of encouragement comes from the old friend who says, "Oh, I had that operation 29 years ago, dear."

Cancer is, of course, a serious disease. It confronts us with the fact of our own mortality, a truth most people keep pushed into the back of their minds. But at the same time, we should keep in mind that even with recurrence or metastasis, women continue for many years to live useful, happy lives.

"It is part of the cure to wish to be cured."
SENECA, Roman Philosopher

After Surgery

What about feelings?

It is important to remember that different women react in different ways to breast cancer. It also helps to know that denial, anger or frustration, depression, a sense of mourning, and fear all are natural reactions— feelings shared to a greater or lesser extent by all of us who cope with mastectomy. They are not feelings to be ashamed of or to try to carry alone.

You may worry about your husband's reactions; he may worry about yours. This is to be expected—and it can be handled in the same ways you handle other problems in your marriage. The more openness you can manage—with kindness—the better. This is a time to make a real effort to keep lines of communication open with the ones you love. You need it and they need it. Withdrawal at this time can be particularly painful for any of you. It may be that husband, family, and friends, reading this booklet can help to establish a common ground of communication. Your loved ones also are undergoing a difficult time, more difficult than we sometimes stop to realize. You may find that facing a problem together brings new understanding and a closer bond to a relationship. Things you once took for granted take on new meaning.

It helps to know you are not alone—and *many, many women are living active and satisfying lives long after treatment.* On a personal level, the Reach to Recovery volunteer from the American Cancer Society can bring reassurance to a mastectomy patient. When she visits a patient—usually after, but sometimes before surgery— many practical details such as exercises and breast forms can be dealt with, but an even more important part of the visit is the emotional support from seeing and talking with a woman who also has had surgery.

If you feel you need information or assistance in handling a problem, phone the American Cancer Society for helpful resources.

Other members of the medical team also can help— nurses and social workers—as can other special sources such as NCI. Again, Reach to Recovery volunteers who have had a mastectomy, and women who have chosen an alternative, can be sources of information. They can provide assistance or find it for you. (See pages 53-60 for sources.)

If you need help, reach out for it.

What special care should I give my arm?

Some surgeons believe no special care is needed, except for exercises, unless you've had the classical Halsted radical. Swelling of the arm (lymphedema) is not unusual, however, after the modified radical or even simple mastectomy. This can be due to possible injury to the lymphatic system necessitated by the surgery. Therefore, some extra precautions seem wise.

It's good practice to remind all medical personnel to use your "other" arm for blood pressure readings, drawing blood, vaccinations and injections. It can be helpful on long trips to elevate your arm or rest it along the seatback of your car or plane (depending on your seat partner!) for a few minutes each hour. Sunburn, injury or infection on your mastectomy side should be avoided.

Other precautions, such as wearing gloves for gardening, a thimble for sewing, and using an electric razor, pertain largely to arms with lymphedema and are listed in the Reach to Recovery manual.

When will the stitches come out?

This varies with different surgeons...generally from one to three weeks.

How soon should I exercise my arm?

Surgeons differ on the answer to this question. Some want you to start on the first post-op day—or as one put it, "the earlier the better unless you have a skin graft"; others prefer to wait.

Tightness and some numbness in the chest and underarm area are to be expected, and commonly disappear in time.

The Reach to Recovery volunteer from the American Cancer Society, who will visit you in the hospital if your physician agrees, will give you an illustrated manual with information about recovery from surgery and what exercises you can do—with the permission of your surgeon. She can also demonstrate the exercises for you. (See pages 50 and 58) Exercising faithfully is important for regaining full use of your arm and shoulder.

Where can I get information about a breast form (prosthesis)? How soon can I be fitted?

The kit given out by the Reach to Recovery volunteer from the American Cancer Society has information about different makes of prostheses and stores in your area which specialize in fitting. Also, most major department stores have a person in the lingerie department who is trained in fitting women who have had a mastectomy.

A very soft, temporary breast form is included in the Reach to Recovery kit, so you can put up a good front even when leaving the hospital. While some lucky women report they get along fine with a padded bra, others with larger breasts benefit from the added weight of a good prosthesis which balances the weight of the other breast.

Fitting for a regular prosthesis can take place as soon as the site of the surgery is healed and your surgeon says it's O.K. There's no real rush. Don't let yourself feel pressured. You should take time to try several forms; they differ considerably in materials and price. A well-fitted prosthesis—and the one which suits you may not be the same one which suits your friend—can give you comfort and a feeling of assurance.

Your local American Cancer Society may have samples of different prostheses for you to see and feel. These can range in price from several dollars to several hundred dollars. Medicare and some insurance policies cover all or part of the initial cost of a prosthesis when prescribed by your physician.

What about breast reconstruction?

For many women the knowledge that breast reconstruction (*reconstructive mammoplasty*) is possible can greatly ease their anxiety and concern. Reconstruction is generally considered possible after many different types of surgery, though not recommended for all types of cancer. Some surgeons urge caution, however, because they feel that reconstruction makes detection of possible recurrence on the chest wall more difficult.

If a woman wants to consider reconstruction, her surgeon should respond to her wishes, and a plastic surgeon should be called in to consult before her mastectomy. Both the advantages and possible complications should be explained and discussed thoroughly.

Some surgeons feel that reconstruction can be done in certain cases at the time of the mastectomy. Others prefer a separate procedure, with the usual wait being about six months. Some, however, would rather wait two years following mastectomy (over half of recurrences occur in this period) until there is less chance of recurrence or metastasis. Reconstruction is also possible many years after mastectomy.

Essentially, reconstruction involves creating a new breast mound by surgically placing a prosthesis under your own skin and muscle, most commonly a silicone gel or inflatable implant. The "new" breast should not be expected to duplicate the original in all ways and will not match your other breast. Reducing the other breast, or a simple mastectomy as a preventive measure, may be part of the total reconstructive procedure.

Reconstruction can be cosmetically and psychologically worthwhile, and with techniques constantly improving, many women are very pleased with the results. You can contact your local American Cancer Society office for information about reconstruction and current publications; also, you could ask whether a Reach to Recovery volunteer who has had reconstructive surgery is available to talk with you.

As mammoplasty becomes a more accepted and successful procedure, some insurance companies now pay for it. In California, insurance companies are legally required to pay for reconstruction or breast surgery performed after June, 1980.

Points to Remember

What is involved in follow-up?

Regular follow-up—that is, check-ups with your physician to be sure there isn't any evidence of recurrence—is essential after mastectomy or other treatment for breast cancer.

The importance of follow-up cannot be over-emphasized. The best promise you can make to yourself is to make sure that your check-ups are thorough and scheduled regularly.

The purpose of regular examinations is early detection of any local recurrence of the cancer, a cancer in the opposite breast, a metastasis, or primary cancer of other sites, including the pelvis.

The sites where early signs of metastasis are noted most often are: 1) in soft tissue—in the mastectomy area, in the opposite breast, axilla, supraclavicular (above the collar bone) regions, or in distant sites; 2) in the bones—ribs, spine, pelvis, extremities and skull (in order of frequency); and 3) in the lungs.

For the first three years, routine follow-up examinations should be frequent, as 60 percent of metastases occur in that period. Another 20 percent occur in the next two years, and the remaining 20 percent after five years.

After five years, you should still schedule a *regular annual* or *semi-annual* exam. And once each year, right from the start, you should also have a regular physical examination to check for possible problems other than cancer.

Of course, if you note any suspicious signs or pain at any time, you should *not* wait until your scheduled exam, but bring it to the attention of your doctor right away.

As with diagnosis and treatment, follow-up should be individualized, tailored to your own particular circumstances—taking account of such factors as the stage of your cancer, and the length of time since your mastectomy or cancer treatment.

But the scheduling, as emphasized by Dr. Robert J. McKenna, Senior Member on the Commission on Cancer of the American College of Surgeons, should be "regular, not haphazard."

The basic routine followed by Dr. McKenna after a patient has healed is to schedule a check-up every two months for the first two years, every three months for the third year, every four months for the fourth year, and after five years, every six months. This, of course, is adjusted to individual needs.

His check-ups include examination of the mastectomy area, the remaining breast, armpit and neck nodes, and the liver area. He inquires about—or the patient brings to his attention—any symptoms such as bone pain, cough or difficulty in breathing, loss of weight or appetite, headaches, or falls.

Routinely tests such as a multi-phase blood test (SMA-12), and annual chest X-ray and mammogram are included. Scans and other tests are used as indicated. You should also not neglect an annual pelvic exam, and regular pap smear as recommended by your physician or the American Cancer Society.

Sometimes a woman will say she'd rather not think of follow-up, because it reminds her of cancer. It is far wiser to schedule your exams at regular times and then relax in between, with the knowledge that you have done what you could to protect yourself—instead of living with the nagging thought that maybe you ought to be doing something.

For cancer of the breast the risk of recurrence or metastasis continues for many years, and *extra precautions—thorough, regular examinations by a physician and reasonable watchfulness on your own part, including a monthly Breast Self-Examination (BSE)—should continue throughout one's lifetime.*

The five-year mark used to be considered a milestone for cancer "cure," but it is now generally agreed that it is best not to establish such time frames. There is too much individuality in cancer—and in cancer cures.

No one likes to think about the possibility of recurrence. To approach this subject in a realistic manner and to avoid feeling discouraged is difficult, but necessary.

We realize that recurrence or spread of cancer may happen; *we also should remember that it may not.* There are valid reasons for feeling encouraged rather than discouraged.

It is encouraging to know that thousands of women are well and happy many years, even decades, after treatment for breast cancer.

It is encouraging to remember that cancer cells are weaker cells. That is why the body's own immune system usually handles them; that is why radiation and drugs can destroy cancer cells more easily than normal cells.

It is encouraging to know that further treatment is now available and that drugs and machines are being improved steadily as their use becomes better understood.

It is encouraging to know that with regular monitoring for recurrence or spread, using modern techniques and tests, it is now possible to discover any problems at an early point where treatment is most effective. This is why consistent follow-up is so necessary.

So it is realistic to expect the best. It is also realistic to recognize the need for follow-up tests and examinations, and to understand the role of adjuvant therapy in some cases.

Your personal follow-up should stress maintaining optimal health—physical and mental—to help your body combat disease.

Fact is, I'm the same car I always was, except now I have a dent in my fender.

BETTY ROLLIN
Author of "First, You Cry"

What other questions should I ask?

Some questions require individual answers—more specific than this booklet can cover. These are some additional things you could ask about:

Hospital procedures
    tests, visitors, hours . . .
How long
    the operation will take . . .

How and where
  your family finds out how you are doing . . .
How much risk
  is involved in the surgery . . .
What to expect
  when you wake up . . .
How long
  before the permanent sections will be read
  by the pathologist
Post-op instructions—
  showers, deodorants, shaving . . .
Length
  of hospital stay . . .
How soon
  you can return to work
  or your other activities . . .
About hormones
  to take or not to take . . .
  also, the estrogen receptor test . . .

What can I do?

Around hospitals and doctors it's easy to get the feeling that everything is happening TO you. And sometimes it's nice just to relax and leave the doing to others.

But you owe it to yourself and your family to be a reasonably informed patient and to take a part in the decisions and actions that can contribute to your own well-being. How?

Experiences will vary, but here are some pointers based on what happened to me . . .

1. When you make your appointment with the surgeon for a biopsy, ask to bring a family member or trusted friend with you. They can help listen and ask questions you might overlook—and think along with you in making decisions. This is a time you can use some moral support.

2. The current debate about *who* makes decisions puts the question as an unnecessary "either-or" proposition. Decisions are made after a thorough, realistic discussion with the surgeon, your physician or other specialists who may be involved—and only after you have taken the time to make sure you have all the information you feel you need.

   What is to be done needs to be a shared decision, combining the physician's experience and technical knowledge with the knowledge only you and your family have about *you*. Some doctors may be more receptive to questions and participation than others. Both you and he need to feel comfortable in your discussions.

3. Remembering all the things that the physician should tell you, and keeping in mind the questions you want to ask—all at the same time—present a real problem. So take paper and pencil for note-taking, and jot down some of your questions ahead of time.

   Even better, if the physician does not mind, you may wish to use a small tape-recorder. It is not just useful to you in recalling the discussion but can be helpful from the doctor's standpoint—it cuts down on the need for him to repeat information that you didn't absorb at first meeting.

You shouldn't expect to be able to remember everything you're told. Studies show that you're doing well to absorb 25 to 30 percent of what is said.

4. Ask questions! This is no time to be shy. So you might ask one or two "dumb" ones? It's better than worrying and wondering. Continue to write your questions down as they occur to you, so you have them ready next time you see the doctor. Keeps you from forgetting them; saves the physician's time. A small notebook, kept as a log, is better than a lot of little slips of paper; and you have the answers there to refer to later.

   Keep on asking questions until you understand the situation to your own satisfaction.

5. Ask about alternatives. The surgeon who performs the biopsy is expected to tell you what he or she thinks is best for you. What are the other possibilities? You may wish to discuss this further with other members of the medical team before you make a decision.

6. Read. If you feel the need for more information, take time before any decision is made to find some of the sources of information listed in the back of this booklet. This will help answer some questions, and may raise others; be prepared to be confronted by conflicting opinions if you read about cancer. However, if you have any questions, it's better to get them answered before surgery rather than wonder about them later.

7. Don't let yourself feel pressured either before surgery or in the process of deciding about any treat-

ment. This is easier said than done, of course. A competent physician will welcome the idea of a *second opinion* and sometimes will suggest consultation. If you have any doubts, you owe it to yourself to have another opinion. The Department of Health and Welfare puts out a helpful pamphlet* called, "Thinking of Having Surgery? Think About Getting a Second Opinion." Always try to talk your feelings out—during the diagnostic period, the hospital stay, and afterward. Many insurance companies and Medicare now pay for a second opinion.

8 Ask your surgeon about arranging to have a Reach to Recovery volunteer from the American Cancer Society visit you in the hospital. These volunteers, women who have recovered from a mastectomy, can help with practical problems and provide a great deal of helpful literature. It's good to talk with someone who has resumed her normal life and activities. (See page 58.)

9. The American Cancer Society can use your help. Find out which of your talents will fit into their extensive program.

   About a year after breast surgery you may wish to offer your services as a Reach to Recovery visitor, but meanwhile there are other ways you can help.

10. Share your experience. You can help take the fear and mystery out of breast cancer. Encourage your friends to learn the technique of breast self-examination (BSE), and suggest they ask their doctors about mammography.

*For copies of this brochure, write:
Surgery, HEW, Washington, D.C. 20201, or see pages 59, 60.

11. Practice breast self-examination yourself! You can avoid alarm over normal lumpiness by asking your doctor or other health personnel to give you instructions in BSE. The American Cancer Society has an excellent small publication explaining how to do BSE and also has other information about cancer, treatment, reconstruction, etc.

    Also, you should check into whether breast self-examination is part of the high school curriculum in your school district.

12. Unfortunately, you may find that job discrimination exists—either overt or silent—against people who have had cancer. The advice of Dr. Robert J. McKenna, California oncologist who works with the American Cancer Society to end such discrimination, is: "Don't quit your job if you get cancer. If you have to look for a new job after cancer treatment, consider taking a part-time position if a full-time job is unavailable." Temporary or part-time positions can provide the opportunity to prove to an employer that you can do the job. Cancer is not contagious—you do not need to fear "exposing" family, friends or co-workers, and they need not fear being near you.

    Federal and California law prohibit employment discrimination against rehabilitated cancer patients. Contact your American Cancer Society if you have questions in this area.

A FINAL NOTE . . .

Telling people not to compare their operations and treatment is like telling water not to run downhill. But remember always to keep in mind the *many variables that make your case different from all the others:* the different kinds of breast cancer, the different stages at which the cancer is discovered, and finally, the real enigma of differences in each individual's own physical and mental response to seemingly similar disease situations.

You are a person, not a statistic; you are why medicine is not just a science, but also an art.

For More Information

Sources of information include the public library, in the card file under "cancer" and "breast cancer"; book stores; the American Cancer Society; and the U.S. Government.

A word of warning—*don't believe everything you read about cancer.* Quoting from Buddha:

> Believe nothing—
> No matter where you read it
>   or who said it,
> Even if I have said it,
> Unless it agrees with your own reason
>   and your own common sense.

And don't expect the authors you read to agree. Ongoing research and clinical trials with consenting patients continue to bring forth new information and promising approaches to treatment. However, time must pass before we can know the long-term results of new kinds of treatment.

Books about Breast Cancer

Breast Cancer Digest: A Guide to Medical Care, Emotional Support, Educational Programs and Resources, National Institutes of Health, 1979. DHEW

Publication No. (NIH) 80-1691. National Cancer
Institute, Bethesda, MD. 20014. No charge.

*Never Say Die: A Doctor and Patient Talk About Breast
Cancer* by Lucy Shapero and Anthony A. Goodman, M.D.
Combines personal story with useful health information.
Appleton, Century Crofts, 1980. $10.95.

Surviving Breast Cancer, by Carole Spearin McCauley.
Non-dogmatic, informative, and reassuring. E. Dutton,
1979. $10.95.

Why Me? by Rose Kushner. Paperpack edition of Mrs.
Kushner's *Breast Cancer.* Newly updated and revised.
Signet, 1977. $2.50.

*The Breast: Its Problems—Benign and Malignant—And
How to Deal With Them* by Oliver Cope, M.D. A clear
and well-written explanation of the normal functions of
the breast and benign disorders, as well as cancer of the
breast. Doctor Cope believes that radical surgery is "on
the way out" and presents the case for lesser surgery
combined with radiation and drugs, based on his two
decades of experience at Massachusetts General Hospital and Harvard Medical School. Houghton-Mifflin
paperback, 1978. $3.95.

What Every Woman Should Know About Breast Cancer
by Jo Hynes Newman. "A simple, direct guidebook that
provides step-by-step descriptions of what happens from
the moment the tumor is discovered, to alternatives to
breast surgery, and how to cope if mastectomy becomes
necessary." Again, you may not agree with everything
she says, but it's a helpful book. Pro-patient participation. Major Books paperback, 1976. $1.75.

Informed Consent by Jane Cowles. The author presents the case for a woman's right to participate in the decision on the best medical procedure for her. Her case history approach holds the reader's attention but gets rather strained when the bad example is too awful and the good example just too good to be true. However, a lot of good information is packed into the telling, and the 44 pages of appendices and glossary are an excellent compendium, a treasure trove of facts about breast cancer. Coward, McCann & Geoghegan, 1976. $8.95.

I Am Whole Again: The Case for Breast Reconstruction After Mastectomy by Jean Zalon with Jean Libman Block. Introduction by Philip Strax, M.D. What to expect, how to seek the best help, dealing with family and friends. Random House, 1978. $8.95.

Books about Cancer in General

The Lives of a Cell—Notes of a Biology Watcher by Lewis Thomas, President of Memorial Sloan-Kettering Cancer Center in New York. Stimulating and enjoyable short essays which put science, cancer and biology in perspective. Bantam paperback, 1974. $1.75.

Medusa and the Snail—More Notes of a Biology Watcher by Lewis Thomas. More short essays—intriguing and informative. Viking, 1974. $8.95.

The Greatest Battle by Ronald J. Glasser, M.D. Cancer strikes one of four Americans, two out of three families; many tragedies of cancer can be prevented, as a majority of cancers may be caused by environmental factors. "It is we who are killing ourselves and our children." Excellent chapter on "What is Cancer?" Glasser writes lucidly and vividly. Random House, 1976. $6.95.

You Can Fight Cancer and Win by Jane Brody, with Arthur I. Holleb, M.D. of the American Cancer Society. The accent is on the positive in this well-balanced and thorough coverage of a wide variety of cancers. With up-to-date information written in layman's language, a medical writer for the *New York Times* helps you to understand cancer and how to take steps to deal with it. Quadrangle/New York Times Book Co., 1977. $12.50.

Understanding Cancer by Steven Leib, M.D. and Mark Renneker, M.D. This book was developed while the authors were medical students to serve as a complete reference on cancer for the average layperson. A comprehensive guide and reference, it has been used widely in courses supported by the American Cancer Society. Bull Publishing Co., Palo Alto, Ca. 1979. $12.95.

Choices: Realistic Alternatives in Cancer Treatment, by Marion Morra and Eve Potts. If you are going to buy only one book, this should be it. Avon, 1980. $8.95.

Medical Dictionary and Health Manual by Robert E. Rothenberg, M.D., F.A.C.S. Definition of medical terms and diseases, with supplement on first-aid, blood tests, diet, immunization and more. Signet paperback, 1975. $2.25.

The Siege of Cancer by June Goodfield. Where we are in cancer research and what the scientists are like who are working on it—human and compassionate telling of their stories by a science writer. Random House, 1975. $10.00.

The Body Is the Hero by Ronald J. Glasser, M.D. The body's immune system—the way the body defends itself against disease—is the product of a billion years of development. Glasser makes it read like a suspense "thriller," including the stories of the discoverers, from men like Semmelweis and Pasteur up to today's researchers. Good chapter on "Cancer." Random House, 1976. $8.95.

The Wayward Cell: Cancer, Its Origins, Nature, and Treatment by Victor Richards, M.D. Second edition. This is a widely used book which presents the main facts known today about cancer. It is directed to those willing to make a modest effort to understand the biology of cells and to scientists who do not specialize in the study of cancer. It is divided into four sections on the biology of the cell, the history and origins of cancer, treatment, and psychosocial problems. University of California Press, 1978. $12.50.

A Comprehensive Guide for Cancer Patients and Their Families by Ernest H. Rosenbaum, M.D., et al. As the title implies, this is a patient (and family) education manual, covering such topics as the role of the mind and stress in cancer and its treatment, nutrition, physical rehabilitation, sexuality, and dealing with hospital procedures and going home. Bull Publishing Co., Palo Alto, Ca., 1980. $12.95.

Late editions of home medical books, such as "Modern Home Medical Advisor," edited by Morris Fishbein, M.D., also answer basic questions about the body and disease.

American Cancer Society

The American Cancer Society is a national voluntary health organization of 2.3 million people united to fight cancer in three ways:

Research aimed at the ultimate control of cancer;

Education for the public and for medical and health professionals; and

Service and rehabilitation for patients and their families, including a cancer information service, equipment, transportation, volunteer visitors and other help. Some local offices provide short-term counseling, and offices can generally refer you to a resource.

Your local Cancer Society, listed under "American Cancer Society" in the phone book, is a source of information about breast cancer; and more important, you always have a friend to advise and guide you there. A phone call is all you have to do to find out about the services and publications the American Cancer Society has which may help *you.*

Reach to Recovery, mentioned earlier, is an ACS supportive service for women who have had breast surgery. This rehabilitation program was founded by Terese Lasser, who realized after her own mastectomy how much women need reassurance and information from others who have recovered from this experience. These women, who are screened and trained, visit either in the hospital or in the home and bring a gift kit containing the Reach to Recovery manual, a temporary breast form, a list of prostheses, and other helpful information.

Other publications from ACS include:

"Facts on Breast Cancer," #2003-LE

"Facts on Cancer Treatment," #2650-LE

"Cancer and Chemotherapy," #6851.00

"Nutrition for Patients Receiving Chemotherapy & Radiation Therapy," #4503.00

"Cancer Facts and Figures" (issued annually)

"Rehabilitation of the Breast Cancer Patient," #3329.00

"How to Examine Your Breasts," #2075—LE

All ACS publications and services are free, and are supported by contributions from the public.

National Cancer Institute

The National Cancer Institute in Bethesda, Maryland, an agency of the United States Government, conducts research and provides grants for cancer research at university medical centers and other non-federal institutions.

Single copies of publications available from the Institute are sent without charge from the Office of Cancer Communications, NCI, Bethesda, MD. 20014.

Some pertinent NCI publications are:

Science and Cancer by Michael B. Shimkin, M.D. For "the informed reader outside the scientific community," this booklet describes the nature of cancer, its effects, treatment and research. Revised in 1973. (NIH) 75-568.

Treating Cancer. Answers some of the often asked questions about diagnosing cancer, surgery, radiation, and chemotherapy. Reprinted in 1976. (NIH) 76-210.

Breast Cancer Digest, 1979. (NIH) 80-1691. See page 53.

Chemotherapy and You, 1977. (NIH) 77-1136.

In addition, NCI funds a toll-free telephone inquiry system, the Cancer Information Service (CIS), which supplies information about cancer to the general public, cancer patients and their families, and health professionals. To find the number for your area, consult the telephone directory or directory assistance. If no CIS number is listed, call the national toll-free service information operator: 800-555-1212 for area office number, or 800-638-6694, the national CIS number.

Under-standing the Language . . . a glossary

Medical terminology, like the "in" language of many groups—physicists, waitresses, all sports writers—sometimes seems perversely designed to confuse the outsider.

However, it does serve a purpose as a sort of verbal shorthand, often saying with precision what would otherwise take more time and extra words.

ADJUVANT THERAPY Treatment given in addition to some other treatment (i.e., chemotherapy is adjunctive to mastectomy). See page 27.

AXILLA The armpit; contains lymph nodes and channels, blood vessels, muscle and fat. Women have a varying number of nodes; 20–25 are usually checked for the pathology report.

BENIGN Not cancerous; not malignant. The two main types of benign disease of the breast are fibroadenoma and fibrocystic disease, really not a "disease" but a hormonal effect. Opinions differ as to whether risk of cancer is greater after evidence of benign lumps, but regular and careful check-ups are wise. A detailed discussion of benign disorders can be found in Dr. Oliver Cope's book. See page 54.

BILATERAL Both sides

BIOPSY The surgical removal and microscopic examination of a piece of tissue by a pathologist to determine diagnosis. See pages 9 and 10.

BREAST Mammary gland. General information about the breast is found in several books in the glossary, especially Dr. Oliver Cope's book, page 54.

BREAST CANCER Many types of breast cancer can be distinguished by the pathologist, some more serious than others, because the cells of different cancers double at different rates and some are less prone to spread (metastasize) than others. The prognosis or course of a disease varies with each individual; we do *not* all react in the same way. A number of factors can influence your individual reaction to disease, among them, the stage at which the cancer is discovered, your state of health and your individual biological make-up.

This list includes the principal kinds of breast cancer. Within these categories, there are many subgroups:

Paget's disease is a carcinoma of the nipple which looks like eczema or scaliness. No lump may be evident until it grows. True Paget's disease is always associated with ductal cancer. It is generally noticeable while still quite small. It accounts for less than one percent of all breast cancers, and generally has an excellent prognosis.

Non-infiltrating carcinoma of the mammary ducts (the channels which carry the milk) is cancer in situ (pronounced "sigh-too")—meaning non-invasive. As more tumors are now found and biopsied when very small, this type of cancer becomes more common. Until recently this form was less than one percent of breast cancers, but is now five percent in some hospitals.

Infiltrating ductal carcinoma is the most common type of breast cancer, accounting for about 80 percent of all such cancers. With negative (normal) nodes, its prognosis is better than with positive (cancerous) nodes.

Medullary carcinoma, named for the pathological term based on its appearance, accounts for five percent of breast cancers.

Colloid carcinoma, also a pathological term, occurs about one percent of the time and has better than average prognosis.

Carcinoma of the mammary lobules, also called lobular carcinoma, is the one which is often both multicentric (having many scattered cells) and bilateral (appearing in both breasts). The lobes are segments of the breast and each is an independent milk gland. It is often found *in situ* and in such cases is 100 percent curable.

Inflammatory carcinoma is a very rare form of breast cancer indicated by redness and swelling or hardness of the breast. These symptoms should never be ignored, as this is a serious form of breast cancer. It is best diagnosed by a skin and tissue biopsy.

BSE (Breast Self-Examination) Inspection and paltation of breasts by the woman herself.

CANCER (CA) A group word that includes some 300 recognized diseases, having in common cells which grow in unrestrained fashion, can invade new body structures and sometimes spread to distant parts of the body, and appear different from normal cells under the microscope.

Within the term CANCER, these are terms used to describe many separate diseases—

Carcinoma: a solid, malignant tumor originating in the lining (epithelial) cells of organs; can occur in almost any structure of the body. 80–90 percent of cancers are carcinomas; most breast cancers are carcinomas.

Sarcoma: a solid, malignant tumor growing from connective tissues, such as cartilage, fat, muscle, bone. Often highly malignant, but only about two percent of all cancers are sarcomas.

Leukemia: cancer of the organs that form the blood, such as lymph nodes and bone marrow; about four percent of all cancers are leukemia. (Characterized by a marked increase in leukocytes—white blood cells.)

Lymphoma: tumor composed of lymph node tissue, from an abnormal prodution of immature lymphocytes—a form of white blood cells; represents about five percent of all cancers, notably Hodgkin's disease.

CBC (Complete blood count) A series of blood tests which can vary as to what is included, but commonly includes white blood cell count (normal 5,000 to 10,000 per cubic millimeter), red blood cell count (normal 4.2 to 5.5 million per cubic millimeter), platelet count (normal 180,000 to 350,000 per cubic millimeter), hemoglobin count—a protein found in red blood cells (female normal 12 to 14 grams), among others.

CELL All living tissue is made up of cells, the smallest unit capable of carrying on the essential life processes—reproduction (mitosis) and production of energy (metabolism). "Cyte" = cell, as in cytology, lymphocyte.

CHEMOTHERAPY Treatment of disease by chemicals acting as drugs. May be administered orally or by injection.

CHRONIC Lasting a long time. Not acute.

CLAVICULAR Pertaining to the collar-bone.

CYST Sac-like structure filled with fluid.

DOUBLING TIME The growth rate of a tumor is expressed in terms of the time it takes to double in size. A single cell requires 30 doublings to reach 1 cm or noticeable size—a billion cells. Cancers vary in doubling time from 8 to 600 days, averaging 20 to 100 days. Thus, a cancer may be present for many years before it is detectable.

DUCTS The channels in the breast that convey milk to the nipple.

EDEMA Accumulation of fluid in the tissues causing swelling. Edema of the arm can occur after radical mastectomy, due to damage or blockage of the lymph channels.

ESTROGEN Female hormone made in the ovaries that affects the generative organs and the breast; made up of estradiol, estrone and estriol.

ESTROGEN RECEPTOR TEST (ER Assay) Some tumors depend on certain hormones for their growth. This test, also called hormone assay, can be done at the time of surgery on the cancer tissue to determine whether changing the hormone environment would be helpful—by removing estrogens or estrogen-producing organs. (See page 29.) Also sometimes referred to as Estrogen Receptor Protein (ERP).

FIBROADENOMA Benign breast disease, usually a single solid tumor of fibrous and glandular tissue.

FIBROCYSTIC DISEASE A benign breast condition common in about eight out of ten women, ranging from minute to large cysts filled with fluid.

FROZEN SECTION Tissue removed by biopsy is frozen, cut into thin slices, stained, and examined microscopically by a pathologist for immediate report to the surgeon.

GLANDS Organs which make and secrete chemicals used locally or elsewhere in the body; sometimes used incorrectly to mean lymph nodes.

GST Graphic stress telethermometry (GST)—can be used as an indicator of breast cancer risk. Temperature tests are fed into a computer to determine higher risk patients. Should not be used alone, but in conjunction with physical examination and mammography

HEMO- Pertaining to the blood.

HORMONE Chemical substance produced by a gland, transported in the body fluids to another part of the body where it exerts a specific effect. Hormone therapy is the use of hormones or substances produced by the endocrine glands for treatment of breast diseases. Hormone assay, or the estrogen dependency test, is now generally available and can indicate whether a cancer might respond to hormones. It must be done on fresh cancer tissue at the time of biopsy or surgery. (See page 29.)

IMMUNOTHERAPY Treatment with vaccines that stimulate the immune response. The treatment can be administered for breast cancer in several ways. In one, inactive cancer cells are injected into the top layer of skin. In another, the old TB vaccine, BCG, is applied locally There is also the relatively new substance, interferon, which several research programs are investigating. Still experimental. (See lymph, page 68.)

IN SITU In place; localized and confined to one area; often the earliest stage of cancer.

INTERNAL MAMMARY NODES Three or four lymph nodes beneath the breast bone on each side, which drain lymph from the inner quadrants of the breast. (See page 23.)

LESION Change in tissue structure or function due to disease or injury—abscesses, ulcers, tumors, etc.

LEUKOCYTES White blood cells. The appearance of the cell determines whether it is a basophil, esinophil, neutrophil, lymphocyte, etc.

LUMPECTOMY An excision of the tumor and a small amount of surrounding tissue. See page 25.

LYMPH Clear fluid, containing cells known as lymphocytes, which fight infections and to a degree, cancer. The *lymphatic system* is the circulatory network of vessels which carries lymph throughout the body, with many *lymph nodes* along the way which can trap and kill cancer cells. The nodes (sometimes called glands) which are involved in breast cancer are—in the armpit (axillary nodes); under the breast bone (internal mammary nodes); or above the collarbone (supraclavicular nodes). See page 23. The entire lymphatic system (and infection-fighting cells in the lymphatic system and in the lymphoid organs, such as the nodes, spleen and thymus) are more than a cancer-fighting mechanism; they are an important part of the body's immune system.

LYMPHEDEMA Swelling of the arm which can happen due to blocking of the lymph channels when lymph nodes are removed. It does not indicate cancer.

MALIGNANT Dangerous to life. In the case of a neoplasm, having properties of invasiveness (into surrounding tissue) or metastasis (spread to other organs of the body).

MAMMOGRAPHY X-ray of the breast; a process used to detect cancers not found by other methods, often a year or so sooner. See pages 6, 7.

MAMMOPLASTY Breast reconstruction. See page 41.

MASTECTOMY Surgical removal of all or part of the breast. (See page 20 for types of operations.)

MENARCHE The time of the first menstrual period.

METASTASIS The spread of disease from one part of the body to another. The most common sites for breast cancer metastasis are lungs, liver and bones.

METASTATIC WORK-UP See staging, page 71.

MINIMAL CANCER This term is now used by different people to mean different things and has come to include invasive, but small, early cancer.

MITOSIS The division of one cell into two cells.

MODIFIED RADICAL MASTECTOMY See page 21.

NEEDLE BIOPSY A tissue is withdrawn through a hollow needle inserted into a lump in the breast. See page 10.

NODAL STATUS Normal nodes are called "negative"; cancerous nodes are called "positive." The number and location of positive nodes in the axilla is an indication of the risk of recurrence or metastasis.

NEOPLASM Any abnormal new growth of cells, usually forming a tumor; can be benign (such as a wart) or malignant.

ONCOLOGY The science of tumors. An oncologist is a physician who specializes in the study or treatment of cancer. (ONCO- is a prefix meaning tumor; from the Greek *onkos* meaning mass.) Subspecialties of oncology are surgical oncology, radiation oncology and medical oncology.

OOPHORECTOMY Ovariectomy. Surgical removal of the ovaries.

PALPATION Feeling a part of the body or an organ as part of making a diagnosis of disease. Examination by touch.

PARTIAL MASTECTOMY See page 25.

PATHOLOGIST A doctor who specializes in the gross and microscopic study of tissues.

PECTORAL MUSCLES Muscles attached to chest wall and upper arms; the larger group is called pectoralis major, and a smaller group is called pectoralis minor. See page 23.

PERMANENT SECTION A procedure preceding pathological examination of tissue to produce a definitive slide showing the cells of a tumor. The tissue is fixed for up to 12 hours in formaldehyde, processed in various chemicals overnight, then sliced very thin, and stained. It provides clear definition so that the type of cancer can be determined.

PLATELETS Very small colorless discs in blood which assist in clotting (thrombocytes).

PROGNOSIS Prediction of probable course of a disease.

PROPHYLACTIC (Preventive) Prophylactic mastectomy is sometimes recommended for women who are considered to have a higher-than-average risk of breast cancer. See page 31.

PROSTHESIS Artificial replacement for a missing body part, such as a breast form.

QUADRECTOMY Excision of a tumor, with a quarter of the breast removed.

RADIATION A general term, including X-rays, gamma rays, etc. In treatment of disease, the use of radiation to destroy rapidly growing cancer cells more readily than normal cells. Includes treatment by X-ray ma chine, cobalt, linear accelerators, betatrons. See X-ray, pages 5, 26, and 28.

RECURRENCE (Local) Reappearance of cancer in its original area or the other breast—as opposed to metastasis to a different area.

SCAN A nuclear medicine process* which outlines an internal organ to detect cancer or other diseases. Made by injecting a weak radioactive material into the bloodstream and measuring the radiation given off. The scans used in metastatic work-up for breast cancer are principally liver, bone and brain. A positive scan can be caused by conditions other than cancer, however.

STAGING Classification of cancers based on clinical examination, X-rays, scans, pathological examination—into localized, regional or systemic (metastatic) stages.

SYNERGISTIC Working together. Interacting. Cancer is believed to be caused by multi-factors, acting syner-

*CT scans of the liver and brain are now widely used, often replacing the radionuclide scan.

gistically. For example, air pollution might not by itself cause cancer of the lung for a particular individual. But when combined with an occupation involving exposure to carcinogens, the synergistic action can result in cancer.

THERMOGRAPHY A method of measuring body heat to identify hot spots due to inflammation or cancer; while thermography can alert the physician to the possibility of cancer, it must also be checked by other means, because hot spots can be caused by things other than cancer, and not all cancers produce detectable amounts of heat.

TUMOR A mass, lump or swelling; can be the result of many causes. Often used incorrectly to mean neoplasm. When used in this limited sense, can be either benign or malignant.

TYLECTOMY Lumpectomy. See page 25.

ULTRASOUND High-frequency sound waves are painlessly projected into the breast in this technique for checking the breast for abnormalities. More accurate equipment is needed before this can be used as a reliable detection technique.

UNDIFFERENTIATED Immature, primitive type cells; descriptive of rapidly growing cancer cells.

XEROGRAPHY A photo copy process by which the image produced by an X-ray machine is displayed on a Xerox plate and transferred to special paper. (See page 7.) The accuracy of either Xerography or mammography probably depends largely on the technique of the radiologist and which he prefers and reads best, as there is still controversy among specialists on this topic.

X-RAY A form of radiation. Short-length electromagnetic rays which penetrate through body tissues. Roentgen rays. Used in both diagnosis and therapy. See pages 6, 26, and 28.

Acknowledg-ments

Accuracy and objectivity can be an author's aim but are difficult to achieve in a field as complex and changing as this one. I want readers to know that invaluable advice and assistance have been contributed during the writing of this booklet by members of the medical profession, the American Cancer Society, and others, including my own family and friends. This booklet has come much closer to those aims because of their help.

A grant from the Macomber Legacy Committee of the California Division of the American Cancer Society made possible the initial printing of this booklet and a pilot project to evaluate and refine it. During this initial testing, hundreds of women read the booklet and shared their time, thoughts and experiences. I want to extend my deepest appreciation for their contribution.

Members of the Service and Rehabilitation Committee, the Professional Education Committee, and the Reach to Recovery Task Force of the California Division of the American Cancer Society reviewed the booklet, contributing greatly toward balance and precision in its coverage. Janet Romano, then a student at the University of California, Berkeley, volunteered to conduct the evaluation of this pilot project. For her time and efforts, I am grateful. I also wish to thank Helen Crothers and Catherine Cordoba of the American Cancer Society staff for guidance, direction, and editing, and Elia Warren for preparation of the manuscript.

For all of us, as women who have a stake in understanding the present state-of-the-art regarding breast cancer, I wish to thank especially the physicians who have given generously of their time and knowledge. Early encouragement and assistance were given by Daniel Burdick, M.D., Clinical Professor of Surgery, State University of New York; Bernard Fisher, M.D., Project Chairman, National Surgical Adjuvant Breast Project, Pittsburg, PA; Robert J. McKenna, M.D., Medical Director of Regional Activities, Los Angeles County-University of Southern California Comprehensive Cancer Center; Frank C. Sparks, M.D., Chairman, Department of Surgery, School of Medicine, University of Connecticut; Philip Strax, M.D., Medical Director, Guttman Breast Diagnostic Institute, New York; and Francisco M. Wong, M.D. Oncologist, Riverside Medical Clinic, Riverside, CA.

I also wish to thank the members of professional committees of the California Division of the American Cancer Society and their colleagues who reviewed and commented on the booklet: Sidney Saltzstein, M.D., San Diego; Neil Andrews, M.D., Davis; Donald Tan, M.D., Glendale; Robert Schweitzer, M.D., Oakland; Victor Richards, M.D., San Francisco; Jay Rowe, M.D., Sacramento; William Wara, M.D., San Francisco; John Hartman, M.D., Ventura; Deanne Gottfried, M.D., M.P.H., San Francisco; and Martin Levene, M.D., Boston, Mass.

I owe a special note of thanks to Jacqueline J. Struthers, M.D., Bellflower, CA, my personal physician and co-author, who answered my many questions patiently and thoroughly.

And a final note of appreciation to the Macomber

Committee for providing additional funds to make this booklet possible, and to David Bull, publisher and mentor, who has been generous with his time and pleasantly relaxed in his approach during the several weeks it has taken to get the manuscript in shape for publication.

GUIDELINES

For the early detection of cancer in people without symptoms

TALK WITH YOUR DOCTOR

Ask how these guidelines relate to you.

AGE 20-40

CANCER-RELATED CHECKUP EVERY 3 YEARS
Should include the procedures listed below plus health counseling (such as tips on quitting cigarettes) and examinations for cancers of the thyroid, testes, prostate, mouth, ovaries, skin and lymph nodes. **Some people are at higher risk for certain cancers and may need to have tests more frequently.**

BREAST
- Exam by doctor every 3 years
- Self-Exam every month
- One baseline breast X-ray between ages 35-40

    Higher Risk for Breast Cancer: Personal or family history of breast cancer, never had children, first child after 30

UTERUS
- Pelvic exam every 3 years

Cervix

- Pap test—**after 2 initial negative tests 1 year apart—at least** every 3 years, includes women under 20 if sexually active.

    Higher Risk for Cervical Cancer: Early age at first intercourse, multiple sex partners

---

REMEMBER, these guidelines are not rules and only apply to people without symptoms. If you have any of the 7 Warning Signals , see your doctor or go to your clinic without delay.

AGE 40 & OVER

CANCER-RELATED CHECKUP EVERY YEAR
Should include the procedures listed below plus health counseling (such as tips on quitting cigarettes) and examinations for cancers of the thyroid, testes, prostate, mouth, ovaries, skin and lymph nodes. **Some people are at higher risk for certain cancers and may need to have tests more frequently.**

BREAST
- Exam by doctor every year
- Self-exam every month
- Breast X-ray every year after 50 (between ages 40-50, ask your doctor)

   Higher Risk for Breast Cancer: Personal or family history of breast cancer, never had children, first child after 30

UTERUS
- Pelvic exam every year

Cervix

- Pap test—**after 2 initial negative tests one year apart—at least** every 3 years
   Higher Risk for Cervical Cancer: Early age at first intercourse, multiple sex partners.

Endometrium
- Endometrial tissue sample at menopause if at risk
   Higher Risk for Endometrial Cancer: Infertility, obesity, failure of ovulation, abnormal uterine bleeding, estrogen therapy

COLON & RECTUM
- Digital rectal exam every year
- Guaiac slide test every year after 50
- Procto exam—**after 2 initial negative tests 1 year apart**—every 3 to 5 years after 50

   Higher risk for Colorectal Cancer: Personal or family history of colon or rectal cancer, personal or family history of polyps in the colon or rectum, ulcerative colitis

notes

notes

notes

notes

notes